AF481255

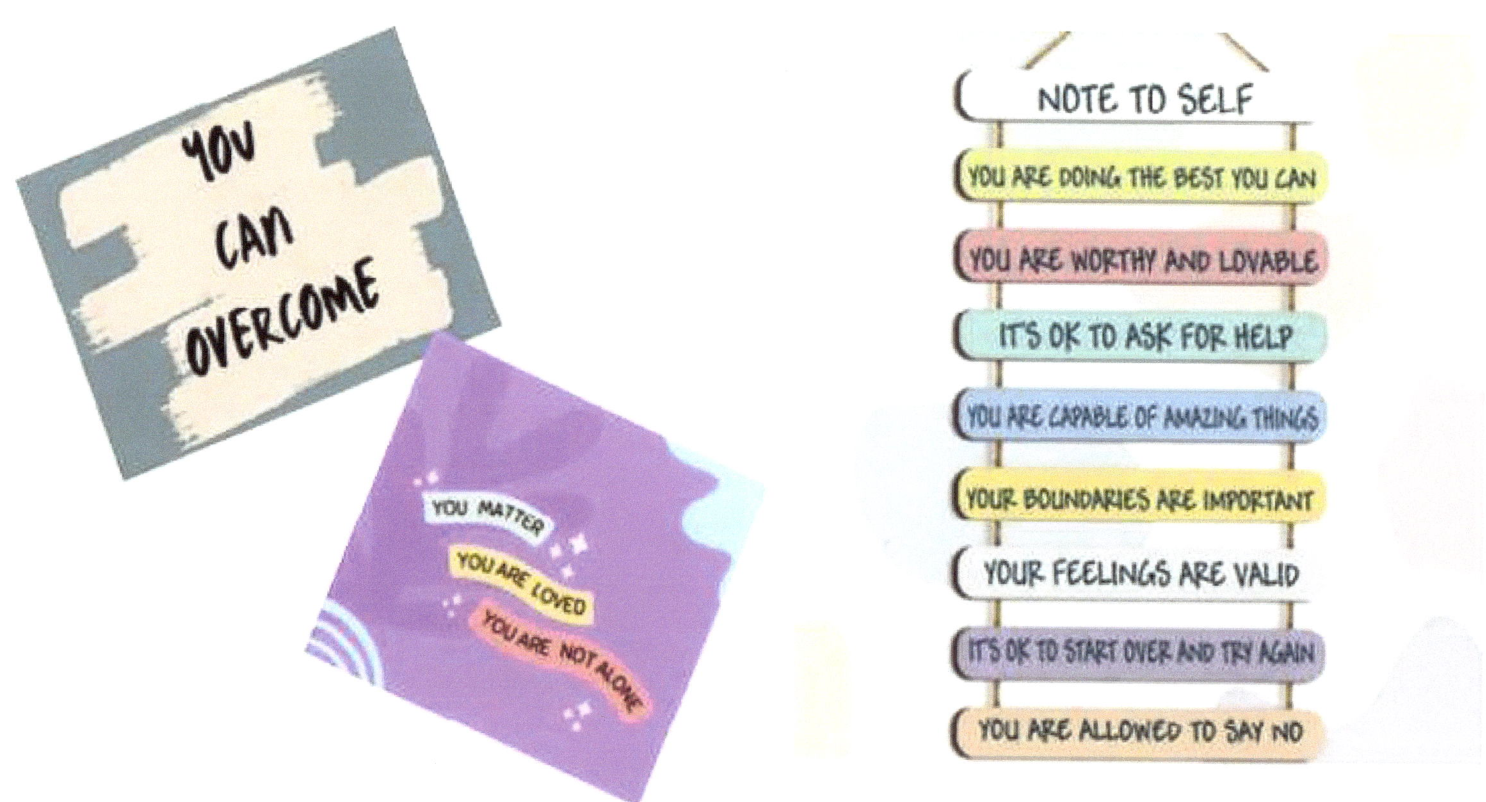

Yeshie's Mental Health Safari:

An Empowering Adventure

Chapter for Adults

Childhood is "supposed" to be a time of imaginative adventures and deep belly laughs. It is "supposed" to be a time when excitement overshadows anxiety and depression is beyond comprehension. Yes, childhood is "supposed" to be a time of playful mischievousness, when we eat dinner and dessert out of order…not a time when which one struggles with an eating disorder. It should be a time when we welcome imaginary friends, not a time to diagnose the strange voices in our heads. Childhood is "supposed" to be a time of health and happiness—free from illnesses of the body, mind or spirit. All said, childhood is "supposed" to be a blissful time filled with butterflies and buttercups; however, trauma can lead to trepidation and mental illness is all too often the youth-stealing consequence of that misdirected creativity.

Few would argue that kids nowadays are growing up faster than ever and their sense of childhood innocence can easily become lost to cell phone screens and fearful dreams. For the sake of introduction I will hold off on reciting any statistics; yet, rest assured that mental illness rates are on the exponential rise in our up-and-coming generation and that the most powerful voice to counter and comfort our youth is yours!

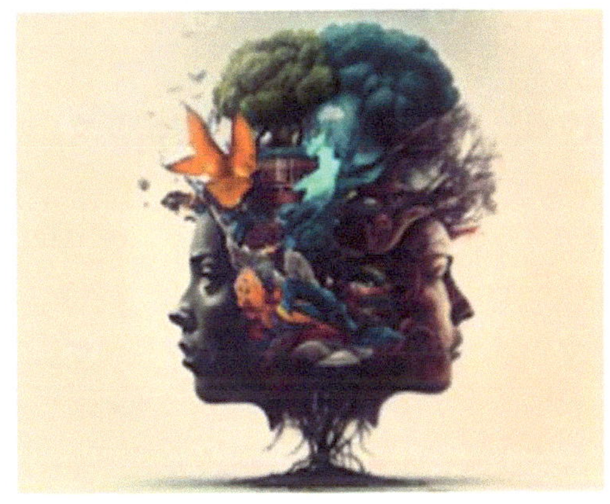

In the story to follow, you and your elementary audience will be introduced to a variety of diagnosis' and disabilities that effect the mind; however, whereas it is incredibly important that youth are exposed to each, it is equally important that they understand that the individual is not the disorder. Mental health problems don't define who we are, they are simply something that we experience at points throughout our lifetime. As Matt Haig writes, "just because you walk in the rain and you feel the rain, you are not the rain." Furthermore, with proper education and awareness, children are able to splash in the playful puddles of "kookiness" instead of sitting soggy in the demoralizing gutters of "craziness."

So how can yours be a voice of health and healing?

It starts by helping youth understand that it is perfectly okay to not feel okay. That its perfectly alright to feel sad at times, perfectly acceptable to get anxious, perfectly normal to be a little abnormal and perfectly natural to not be, well…*perfect*. We all struggle to fit in periodically and we all struggle to understand our feelings and emotions when they run awry. In such, maybe *perfect* is the wrong word to use when speaking about Mental Health because there is no such thing as perfection when it comes to the mind. We are all a little looney on occasion—and that's a good thing because what one defines as *crazy*, another might define as personality.

As you and your kiddo companion flip the pages forthcoming, take time to dialogue about each safari animal that you encounter and, in doing so, you might reference a few contemporary examples of each that are present in your own lives. It may be a friend or family member with autism, a houseless neighbor on the street that yells obscenities or even a pet that is a little over-anxious. The goal is to normalize unpleasant or obtrusive emotions and feelings in a way that assures youth that they are never alone when afflicted by them. As you chat, be sure to highlight the good in each character by pointing out the ways through which each character can have a positive impact on the larger whole despite, or in some cases as a result of, their struggles. For example, a Bi-Polar Bear named Bill becomes a trusted friend, an Obsessive Compulsive Ostrich keeps things clean, an Armadillo with Autism glows with creativity, and a Stuttering Snake named Stuey shares an amazing lunchtime sandwich spread. Every person—or animal in the case of our story—possesses a gift to share in addition to a cognitive ailment to overcome. Furthermore, through openness and companionship, each is able to share those gifts and overcome their Mental Health hiccups alongside new and authentic friends.

Finally, don't shy away from sharing about your own struggles! I promise that your openness will not negatively impact the superhero persona that you hold with your youth, but enhance it. After all, the strongest role models are not the ones who don't struggle, but the ones who aren't afraid to admit it and seek support when they do. Opening up about your own Mental Health ailments allows your children to feel comfortable and confident in doing the same. This willingness to share sets the stage for an honest, trusting and open relationship that will lay the foundation for a lifelong lesson in self and social-awareness and acceptance.

That said, thank you for your willingness to engage in such an important topic alongside your children—and trust that you are not alone on the journey. I hope that you enjoy the tale to follow and that you feel comfortable reaching out at any time with questions, stories, etcetera in regards to the mental health of your family, class or group.

About the Author:

In addition to being an aspiring author and surf-bum in training living in Santa Cruz, CA, Rev. Capt. Ryan Althaus is a neurodivergent minister and nonprofit leader who functions as the regional inclusion affiliate of the National Presbyterian Church. He has a passion for disability and mental health awareness, and has written several books (children's and adult) related to the subject. When not writing or preaching, Rev. Ryan lives the life of a sailboat Captain alongside of his K-9 companion, Rafiki, and you can read all about him and his work via his website: www.thesurfingmango.com.

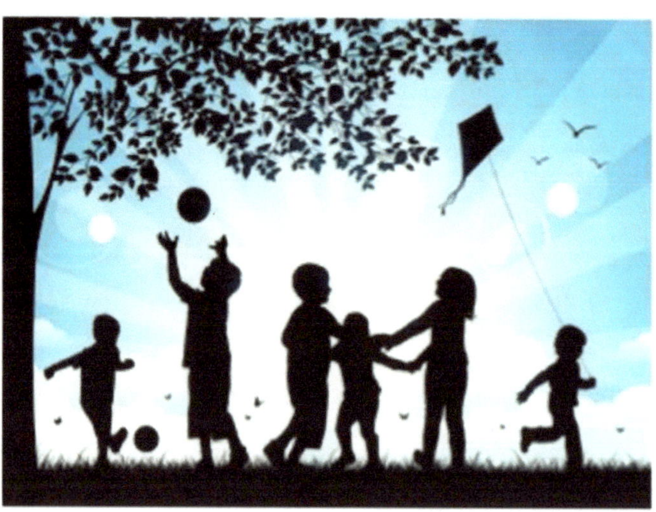

"A Safari! Oh Joy!" shouted Yeshie the Sheep,
After lying awake all night — too excited to sleep.
With monkeys on his mind, he grabbed a banana mid-leap,
As he dashed out the door, towards a big green jeep.

A hippo? A flamingo? A giraffe, zebra, or lion?
Would the first animal he saw be walking, galloping, or flying?
Just no slithering because snakes made him run crying,
or any of the buzzing bugs that kept multiplying!

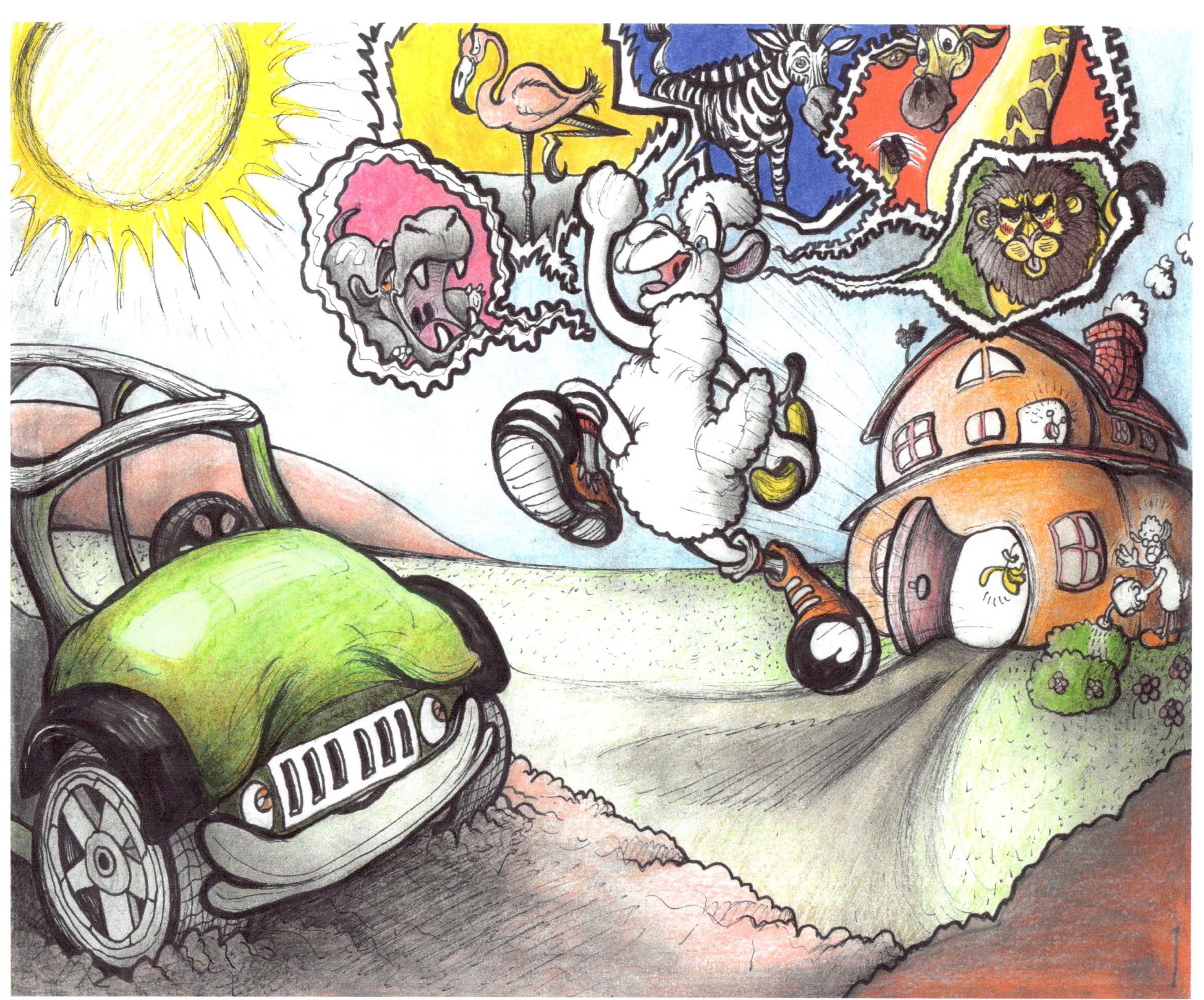

The jeep bounced up and down as it rolled over rough rocks,
And splashed through a muddy puddle, soaking Yeshie's sheep-wool socks.
"What's that?" Yeshie yelled as he pulled a pair of binoculars from the glove box.
Before climbing from the jeep—sly like a fox.

Yeshie cheered when a grand grey creature stepped out from the trees,
whose wrinkly skin stretched from his ears to his knees.
"Who are you?" Yeshie's question caused the creature to freeze.
"Why, I'm Eli the elephant...I think. Now would you help me get home, pretty please?"

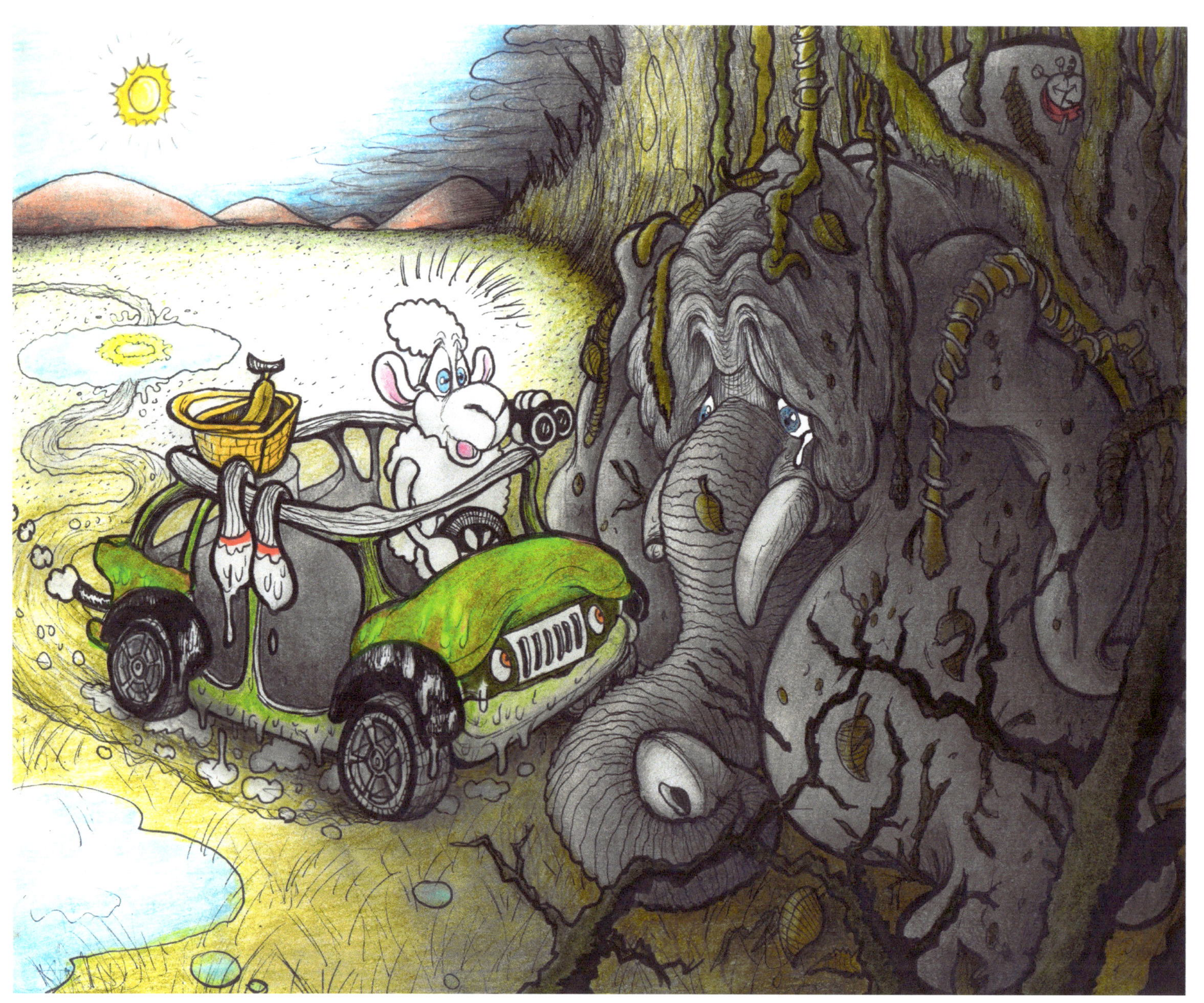

"Of course I will help you," the sheep shouted up towards the sky,
At the trunk of the elephant, as it swatted a fly.
"I cannot remember my way home, no matter how hard I try.
In fact, I forget a lot of things these days," Eli admitted, then
started to cry.

"That's okay, Mr. Elephant," Yeshie said in a soothing tone.
"It would be my pleasure to help you find your way home."
"I'm not crying because I'm lost," Eli replied with a groan.
"I'm crying because elephants aren't supposed to forget things—
so I feel sad and alone."

But Eli was not a failure, and there was no need to feel fitful.
He simply had something called Alzheimers that made him forgetful.
So Yeshie passed Eli a tissue and gave a gentle pull,
on the ear of an absent-minded elephant who seemed super cool.

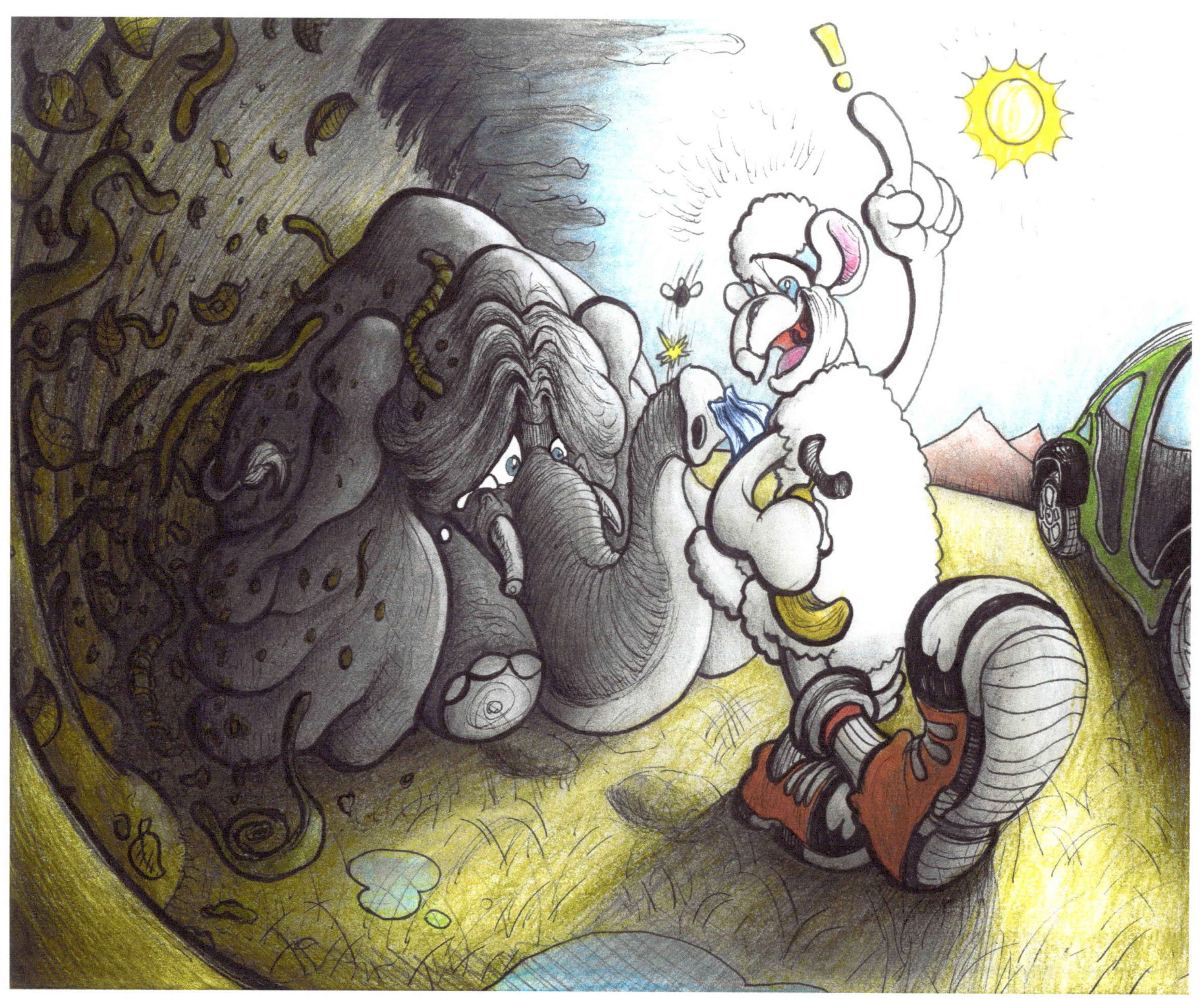

The Jeep was a little small for Eli's elephant sized rear-end,
But that didn't stop Yeshie from helping his new found friend.
"We can walk together beside it!" The sheep's lips started to bend,
into the shape of a smile that he was happy to lend.

Together the sheep and elephant trotted across the savannah,
until they ran into a stripped horse, wearing a red bandanna!
"What's your naaaammmmmmme," Yeshie yelped, as he slipped on the
peel of a banana.
The horse poked Eli with her hoof, then replied: "My name is Ana."

"Hey, why'd you poke me?" asked the elephant of the stripped
horse,
"Why...? Well, to make sure that you were real, of course."
"Real?" Eli feared his confusion must be getting worse.
"Yeah, sometimes I see things that aren't there and hear voices
that have no source."

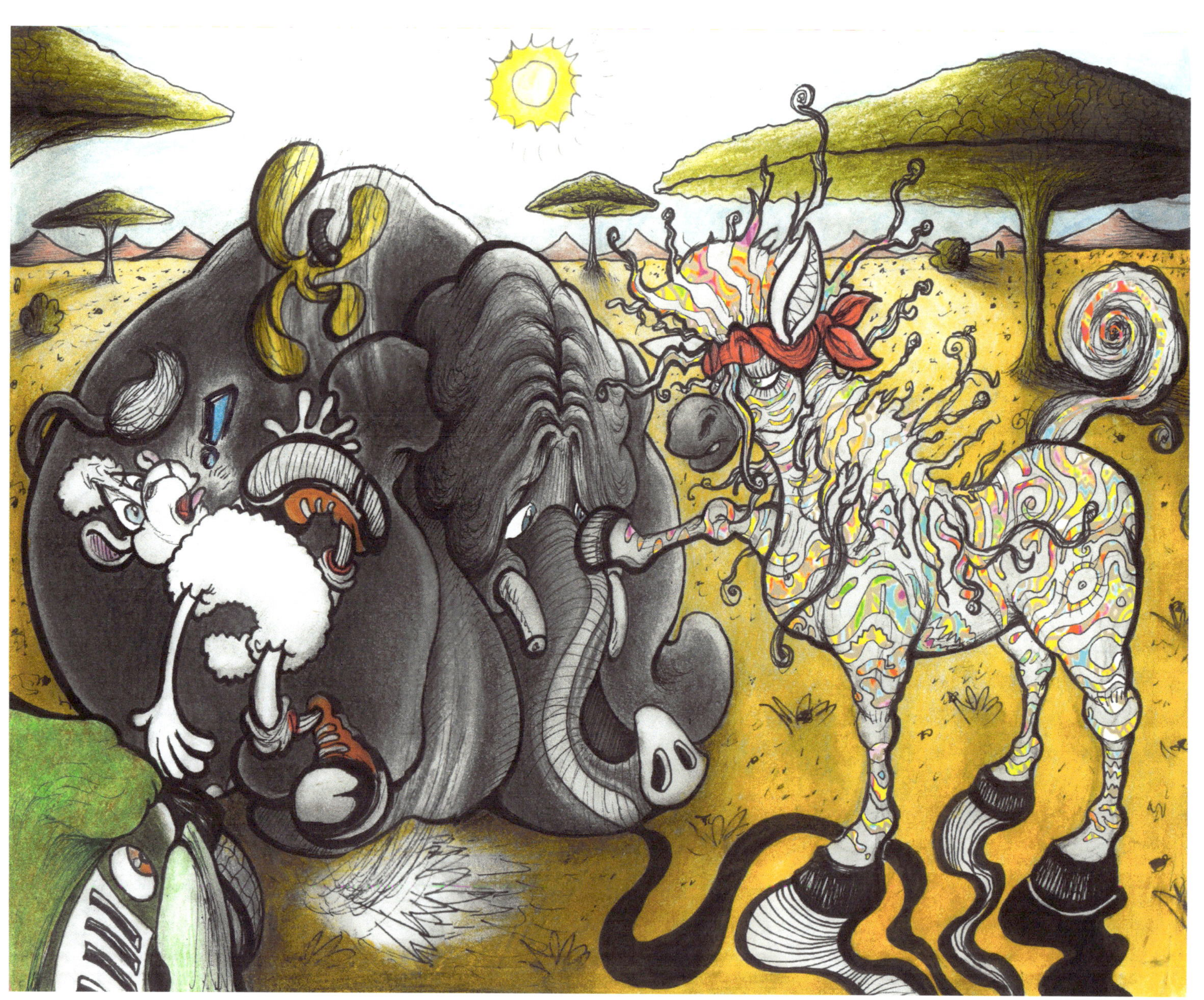

Ana looked sad as she pulled the bandana down over her eyes.
"'I'm a zebra, not a horse," she said. Then she started to cry."
"I have something called schizophrenia-and much like these stripes of mine,
It makes it hard to know what's real or fake," she said in reply.

Ana galloped in a circle, and much like she'd claimed,
Her stripes swirled into spirals while the wind blew through her mane.
Yeshie hated to se such a pretty zebra feeling such pain;
Just because other animals labeled her imagination insane!

"There is nothing wrong with hearing or seeing things that others do not,
After all, whose to say what I call a stripe isn't a poke-a- dot!
However, whenever you get sad or confused, it sure helps a lot,
To have fun friends at your side when through the savanna we trot!"

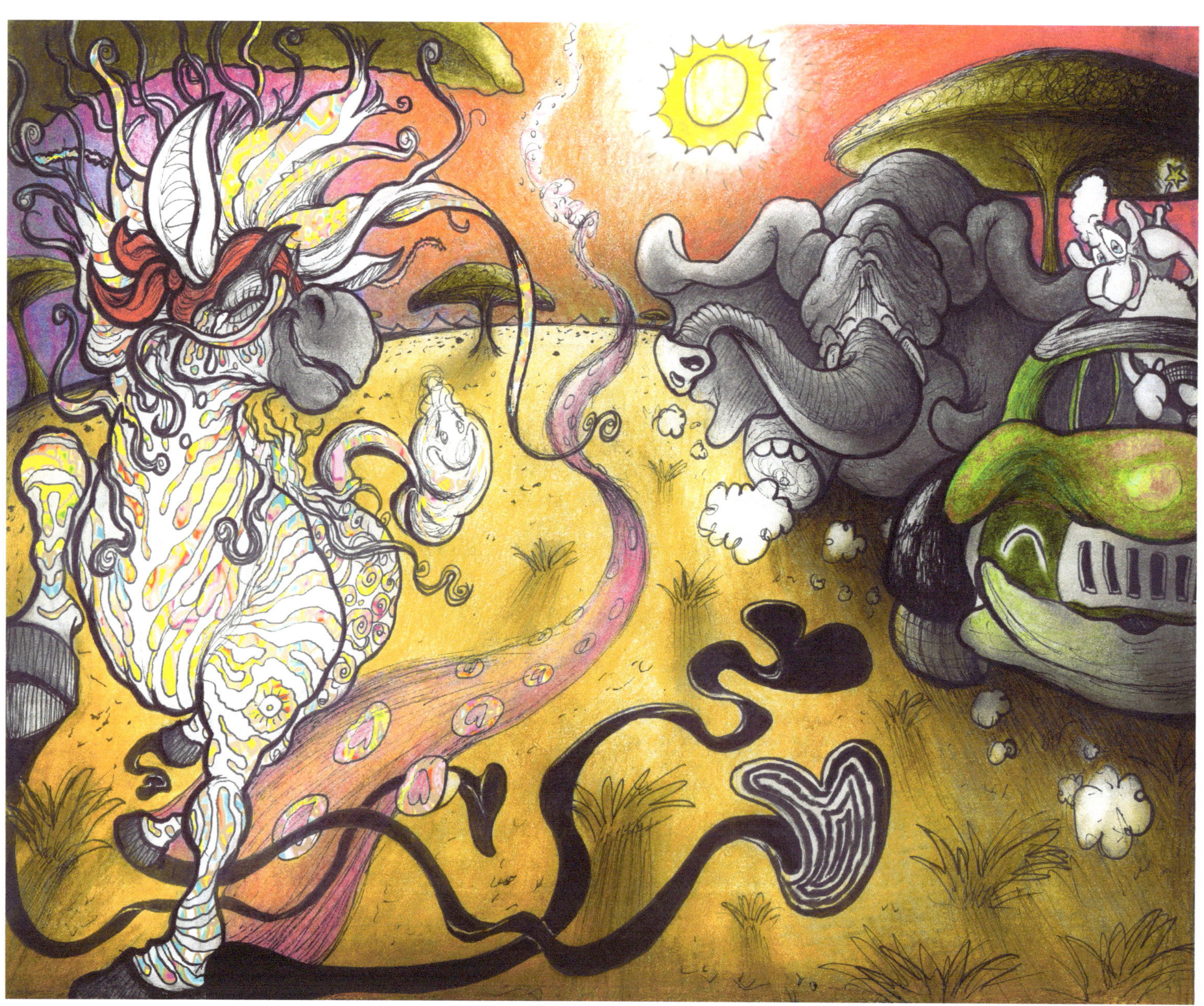

So together the absent-minded elephant and sheep smiled and said:
"Ana, we would love to have a schizophrenic zebra join us as we tread!"
 With those welcoming words that the trio was led,
Across African planes — under skies of pink, orange and red.

The day had grown hot, and their mouths were getting dry,
So the three newfound friends wandered to a watering hole nearby.
 It was there that a great big white bear greeted them with a sigh:
"I am Bill the Bi-polar bear," he declared. "Hello and Goodbye!"

"A polar bear in Africa? I must be seeing things again,"
said the schizophrenic zebra of this 'bi-polar' bear she thought was pretend.
But bi-polarity isn't a bad thing, it just meant Bill's feelings bounced between two ends;
North or south, he couldn't decide, so in Africa he tends.

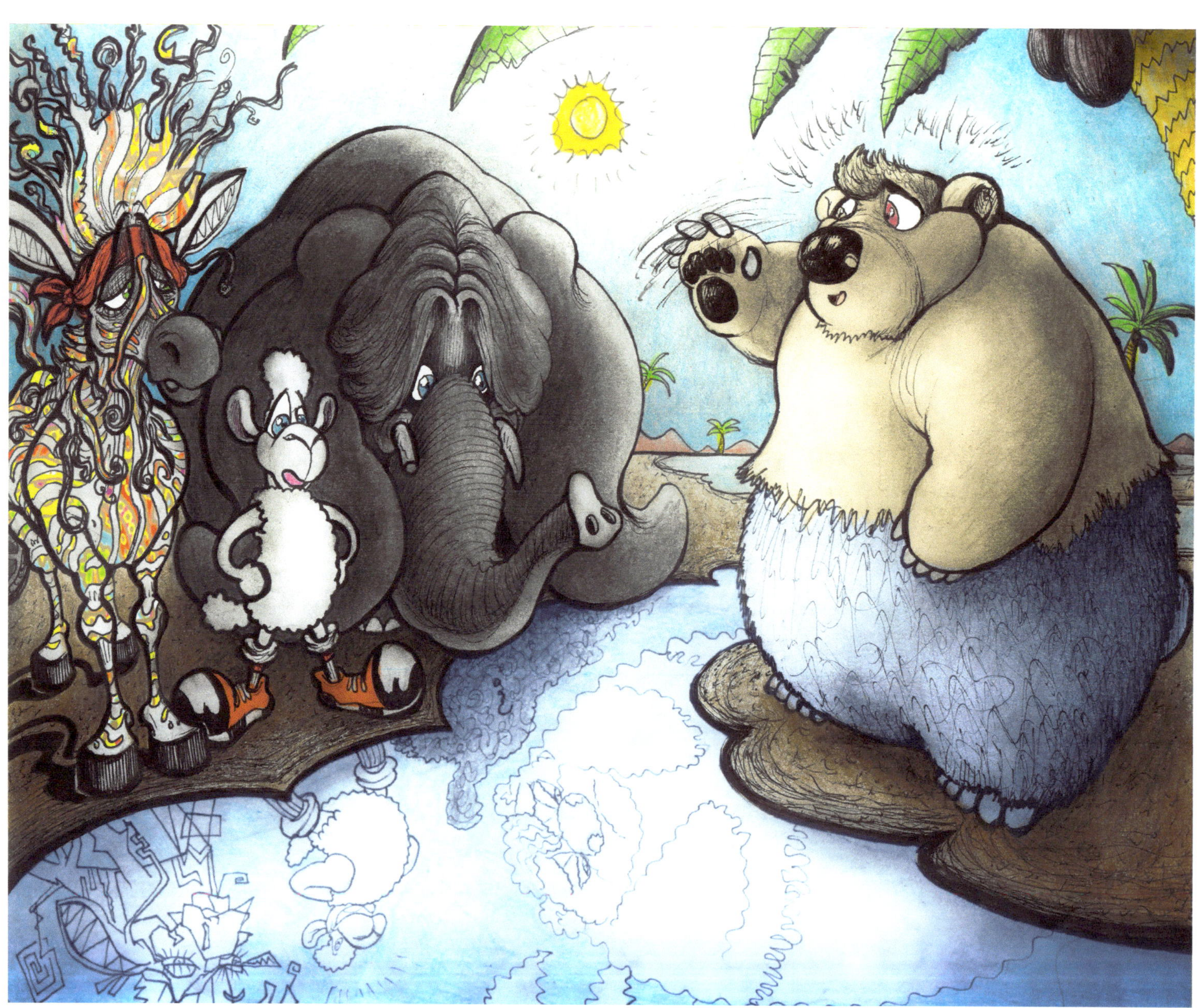

Sometimes I'm extra happy, but happy can quickly turn sad.
But being here at the watering hole always makes me glad!
"'Everyone's feelings change, so don't let your's get you mad,
Because no matter what emotion you are feeling, this sheep thinks you're
super-duper rad!"

Then Bill told the trio about two friends that traveled together:
Maurice the manic monkey, whose energy was better;
Than Dave the depressive dingo whom always seemed to be under the weather.
Combined they called themselves manic-depressive, and they were best buddies
forever!

Although they had not seen Maurice the Monkey, Yeshie thought he knew,
That it was off of his banana peel t h a t , earlier, he flew.
Meanwhile, while the others chatted, Eli sucked up the water blue,
And with his mighty trunk, a sprinkler he did construe!

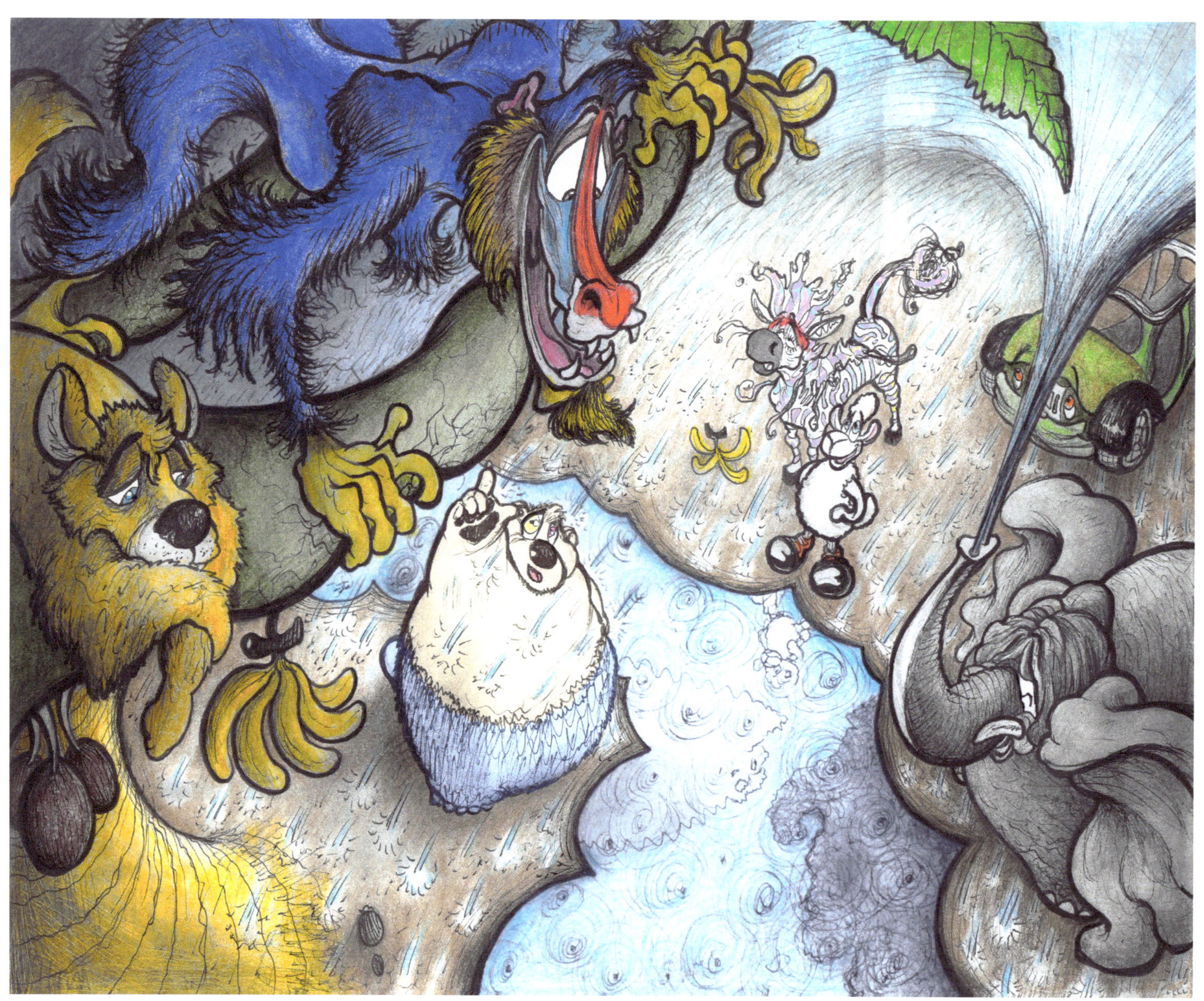

The shower was refreshing, and the gang danced and cheered;
But their merrymaking ended abruptly when Yeshie saw the snake that he
had feared!
He watched as it slithered along the shoreline, dragging a scraggly green beard,
And decided that the snake wasn't scary after all—just a lit the weird!

Eccecccussssse me for intersrerrrrupting," the snake said to the stunned bunch.
"But it just so happens that I packed sssssome extra ssssandwhiches for lunch.
Yeshie was still mer vous, but the group had a hunch,
That this snake was pretty special, so with him they did munch!

"'Thank you for sharing, that sure was very nice!
What is your name," And asked, before grabbing another slice.
"'Sssssssssome call me ssstuttering Sssstuey!" The snake seemed to say things twice.
"And I love to sssssshrare with others at thissss oasissss paradisssse.'"

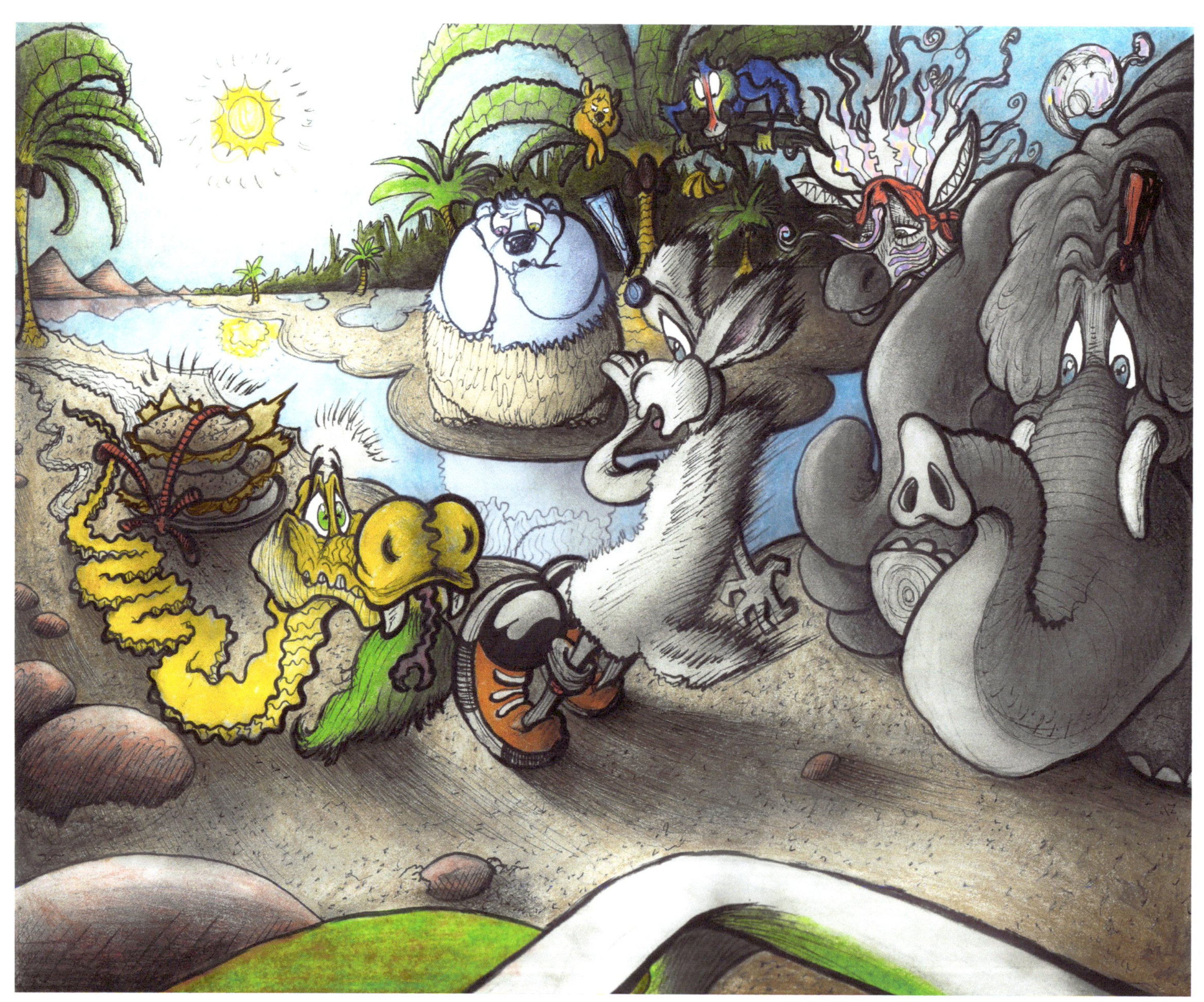

"Say Stuey, you should join us," said the snake-fearing sheep.
"We are on a journey to find Eli's home and there is an extra seat
in the jeep."
"Gosh, that's awful kind, but after lunch I like to ssssleep."
And after waving goodbye, Stuey slithered toward a sunny-stone
without a peep.

The group sure was grateful for the sandwich-sharing snake,
It had been a long morning and their bellies had been begging for a
lunch break!
And despite his stuttering and slithering, Stuey sure knew how to
make,
The perfect peanut butter sandwich for a picnic at the lake.

So with happy tummies the team traipsed onward towards Eli's
home,
Through green jungles they trekked and across golden savannas they
roamed.
Ana paused to kick a coconut, but the bi-polar bear grumpily
moaned;
"We don't have time to play soccer today, Ana" he insisted, in a
serious tone.

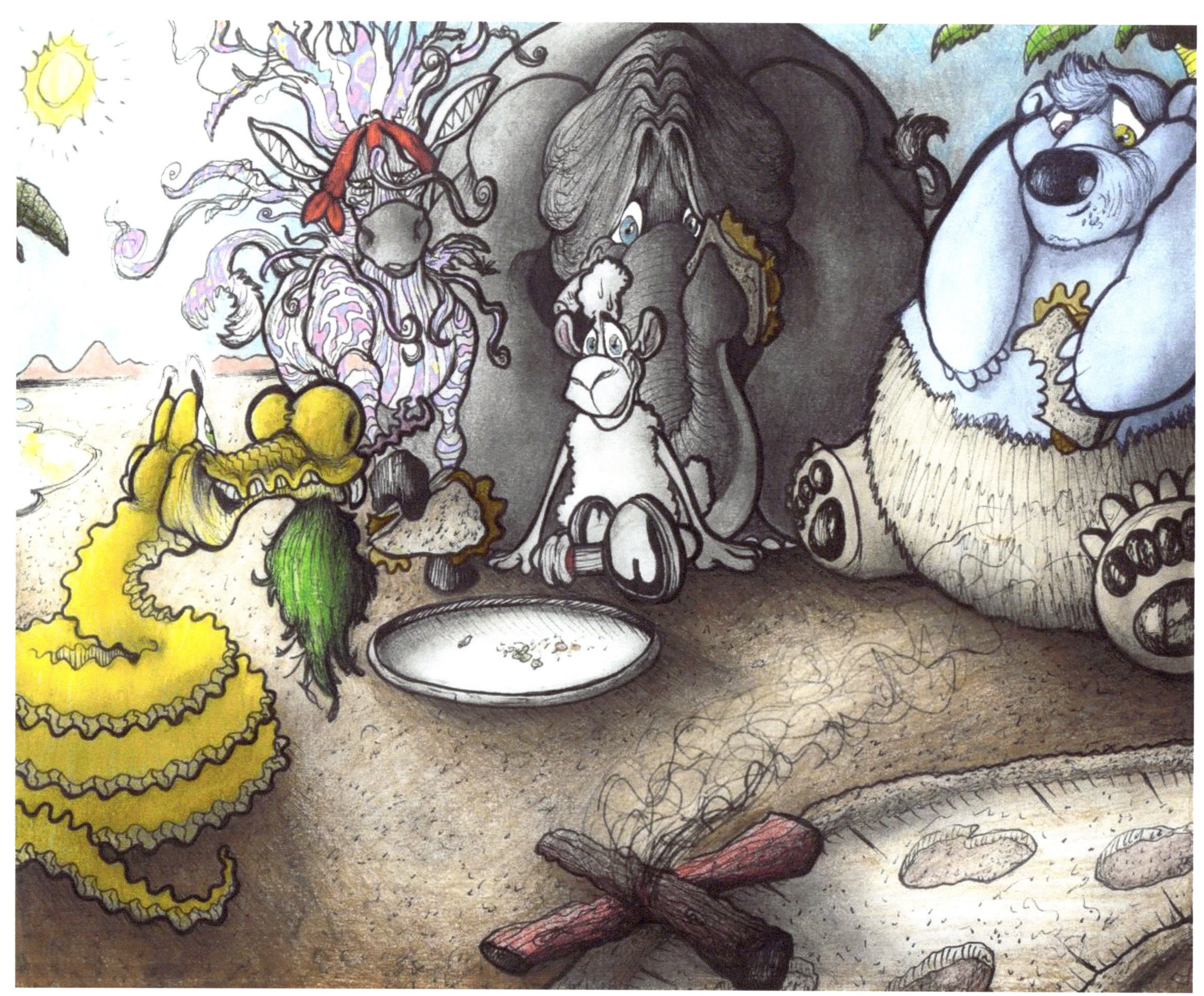

"No time to play?" The schizophrenic zebra seemed confused.
The voice in her head had told her to kick the coconut — but
Bill was obviously not amused.
"Its okay Ana," Eli the Elephant said after taking a second to
muse.
"There is a field by my den where you can play soccer all evening
long if you choose!"

The Elephant sure was exhausted; after all, he was pretty old,
But his enormous ears perked up when he saw an armadillo crossing
the road.
He had never met one of these armored animals in person, but he
had always been told,
That their wisdom was more valuable than 27 bars of gold!

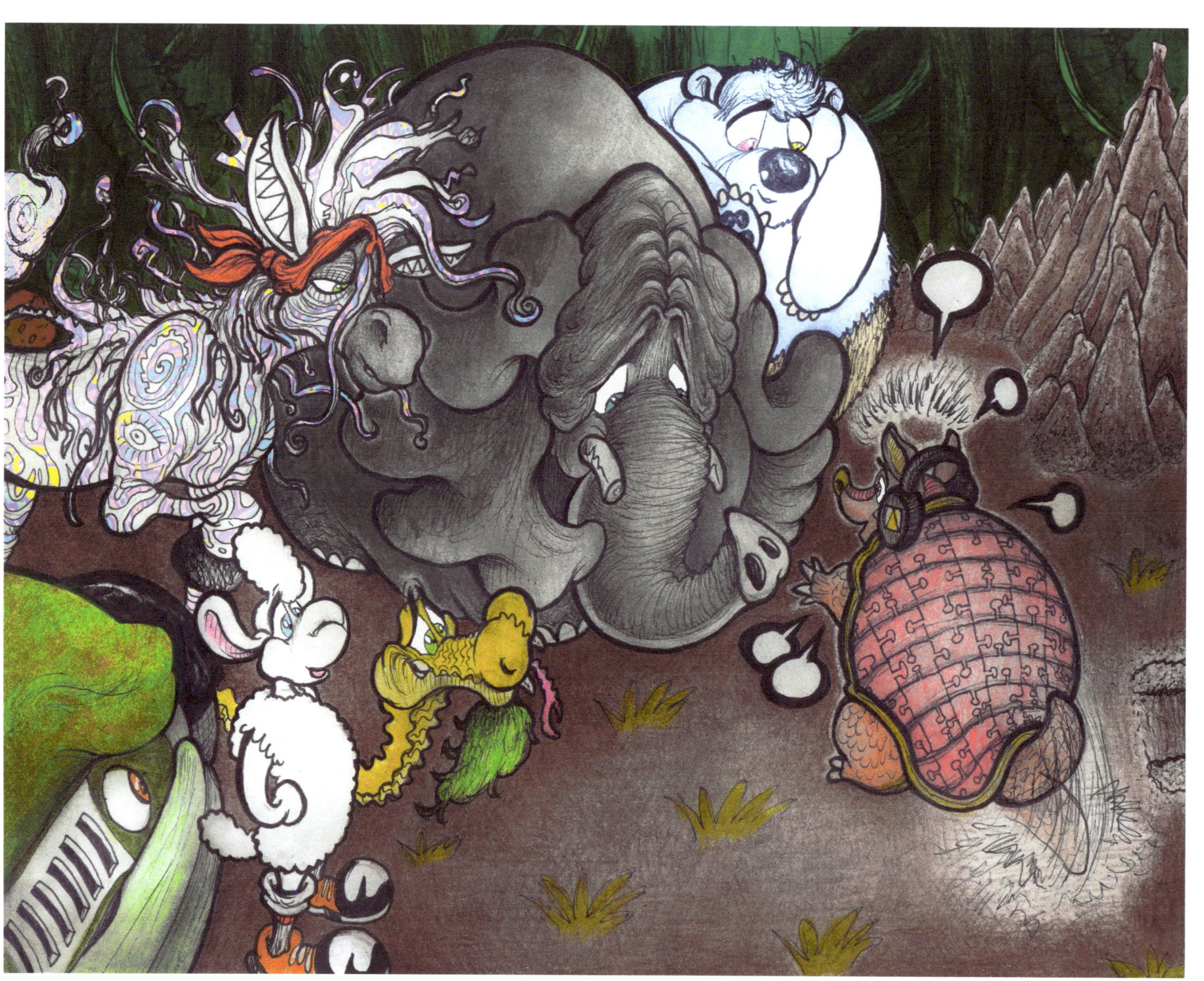

"Wow, Ernie the Armadillo! Autism sure is a beautiful gift,"
Said Yeshie the Sheep, before offering Ernie a lift.
"Indeed, it can be, but autism can also create quite a rift,
Between me and the world—you see, I'm very sensitive to things
that others miss."

"Loud sounds and bright lights often cause me to stay hidden,
Under this shell-like skin that dulls the colorful gifts I've been
given."
"While, I think that you are a hero and deserve a blue ribbon,
For shining so brightly," exclaimed Eli. "Despite being anxiety-ridden."

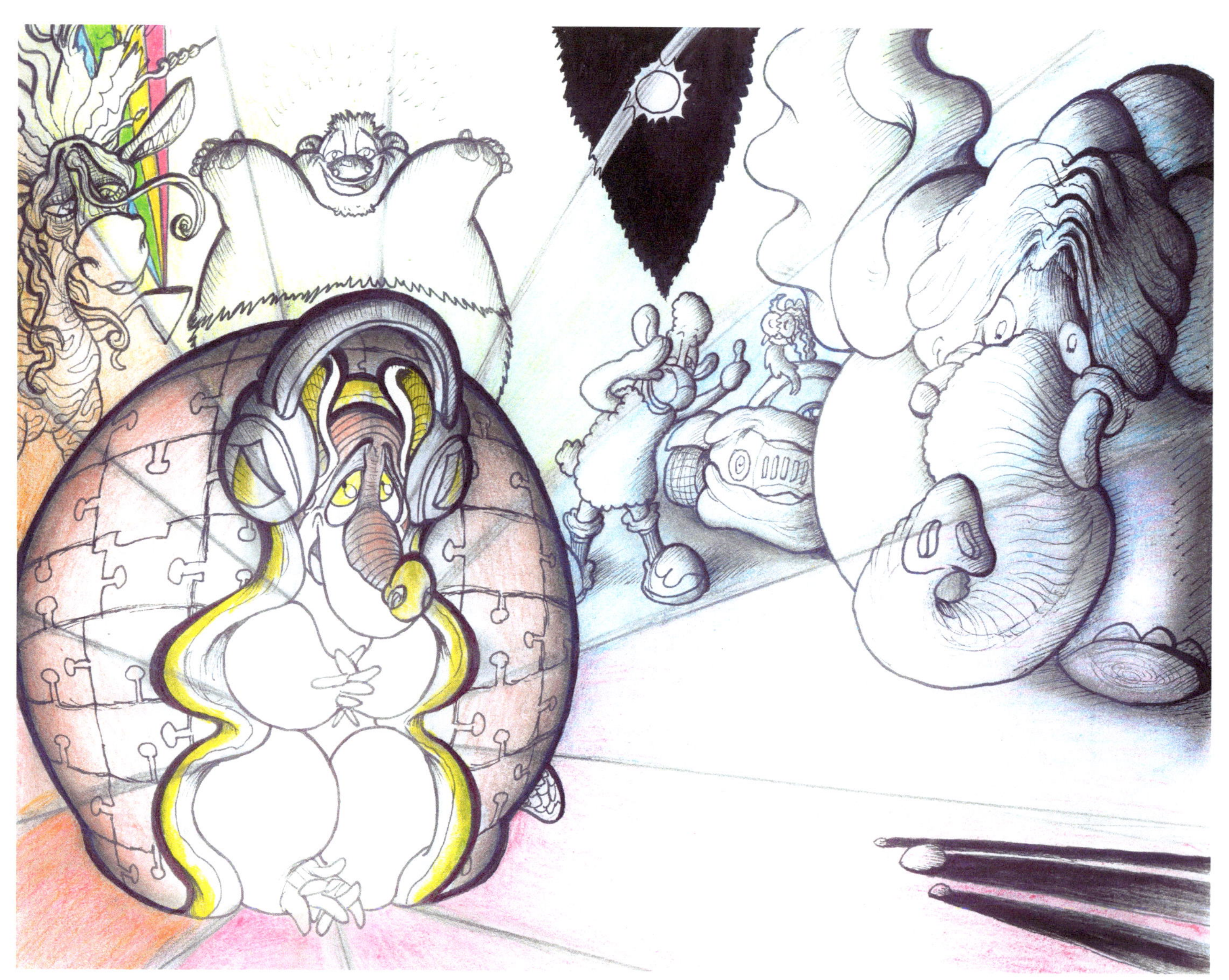

Ernie thanked his new friends, and sent the group on their way,
So they could get Eli home before the sun set on the day.
"Oh, one more thing," Ernie started to say.
"You might pass my friend Paul, a Chimpanzee with Cerebral Palsy,
who loves to play!"

"Oh joy!" shouted the soccer-loving schizophrenic zebra named Ana.
"I need a buddy to kick a coconut with, and I could use a banana!"
With those words the gang strutted off, staring upward at the
rainforest panorama,
But instead of Cerebral Paul, they met a mask-wearing panda!

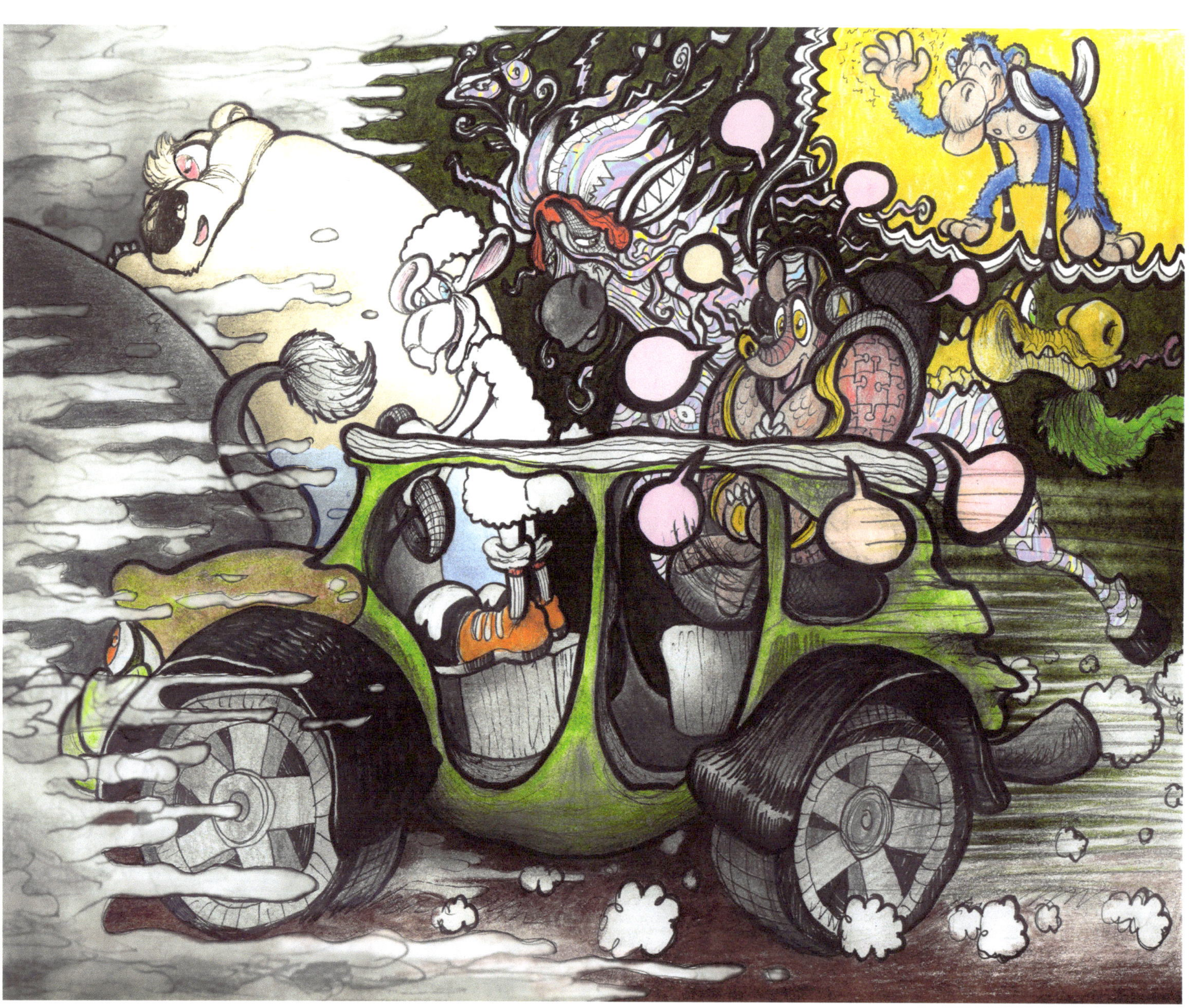

He was there...then he wasn't...then he came into view again.
"Do you need a watch or a wallet?" he asked. "They are free for
you my friends.
My name is Patrick, and I have a problem that you might help
me mend...
You see, I am a kleptomaniac with a conscience—thus I'm pulled
between two ends."

A klepto-what?" Yeshie repeated the word in the form of a question.
"Kleptomaniac—it means I can't stop taking things, like the
watch that I mentioned.
However, I don't like to steal, so there lies the tension,
In fact, I always give back each and every stolen possession.

"Hey! That's my watch," Bill the bi-polar bear shouted with a
bare wrist.
"And that's my wallet," Ana announced, never knowing it had gone amiss.
"How did you do that you do that," Eli asked. "Please, give us the gist."
"I'll show you instead," Patrick replied, before disappearing into the mist.

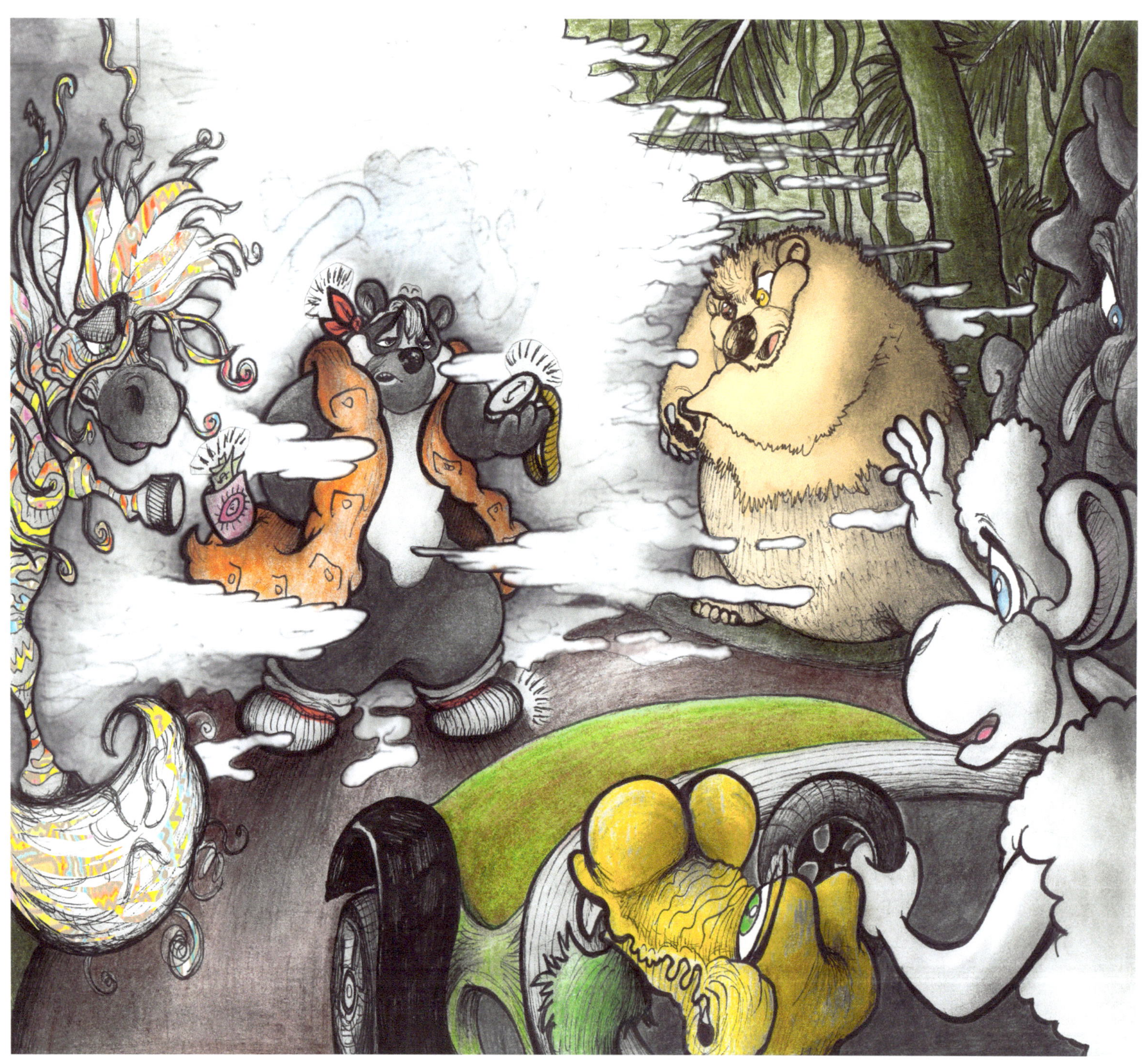

When he reappeared he was wearing Ana's red bandanna and the wool socks,
that Yeshie had received as a gift from his flock.
Then the pick-pocketing panda returned it all—even Bill's watch that went tictok,
Because it didn't feel good to steal, and Patrick feared that in prison, he'd might get locked.

"I sure do apologize," Patrick pleaded for forgiveness,
"It's just...I cannot seem to stop stealing things, despite all of my resistance.
So I fled from the rainforest to the jungle—and now I keep my distance,
from anyone that might be hurt by my criminal existence."

The group of wandering friends listened to the Panda's sad confession.
They liked Patrick a lot, and didn't blame him for his burglary obsession.
After all, stealing was not this masked-bear's true intention,
He just struggled to find a better means of self-expression.

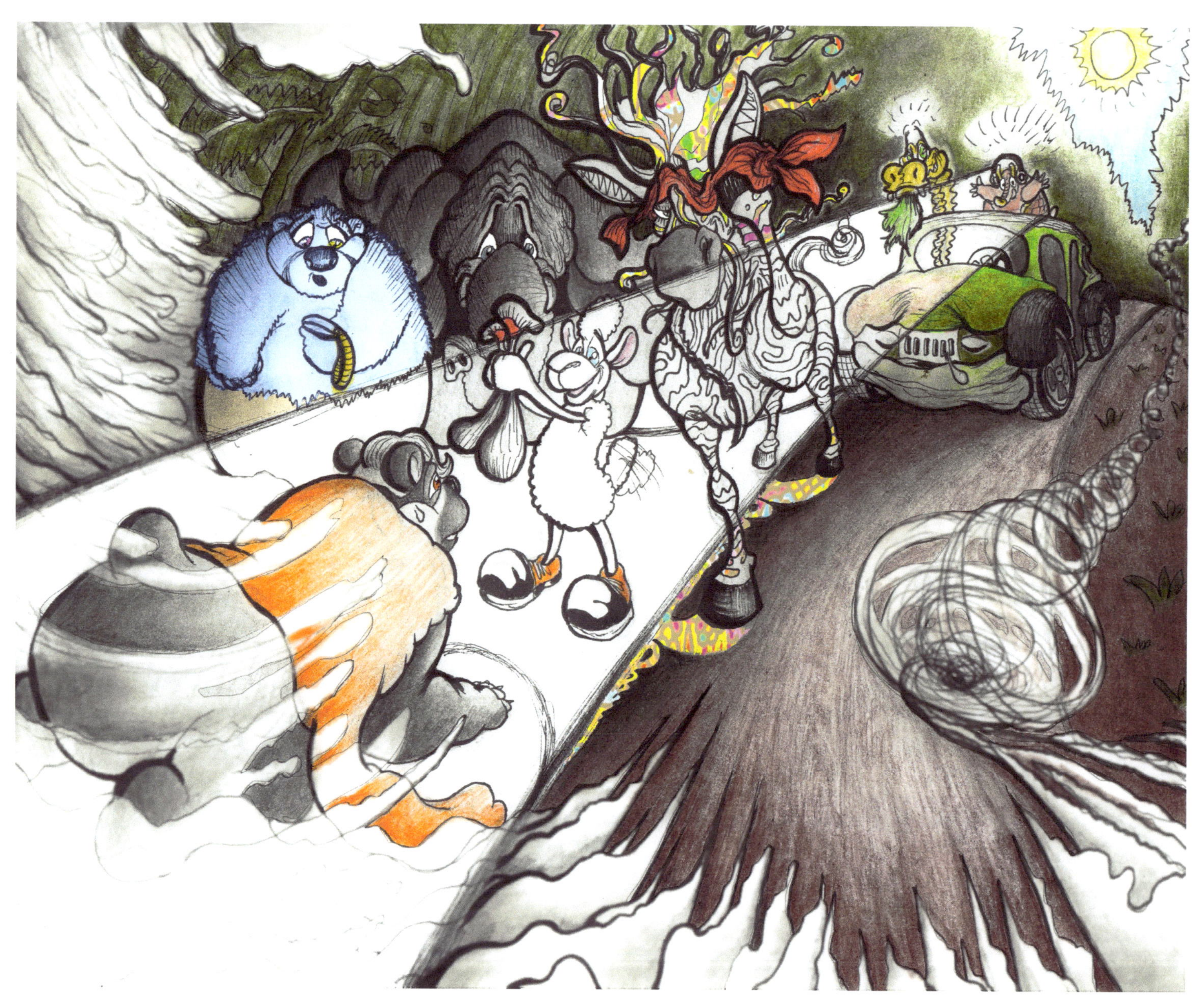

"We all do things that we know we shouldn't do every now and again,
But that isn't a reason to run away from your family and friends.
When you feel like fleeing from those who love you, why not share your
struggles instead...
You may just find, they have support of which to lend."

With those words Yeshie invited the Panda a ride in the big green jeep,
And Patrick happily accepted because the hill up ahead looked pretty steep!
Yeshie knew that Patrick meant well, and that a promise he would keep,
To ask before he takes things, and share any gifts that he might reap.

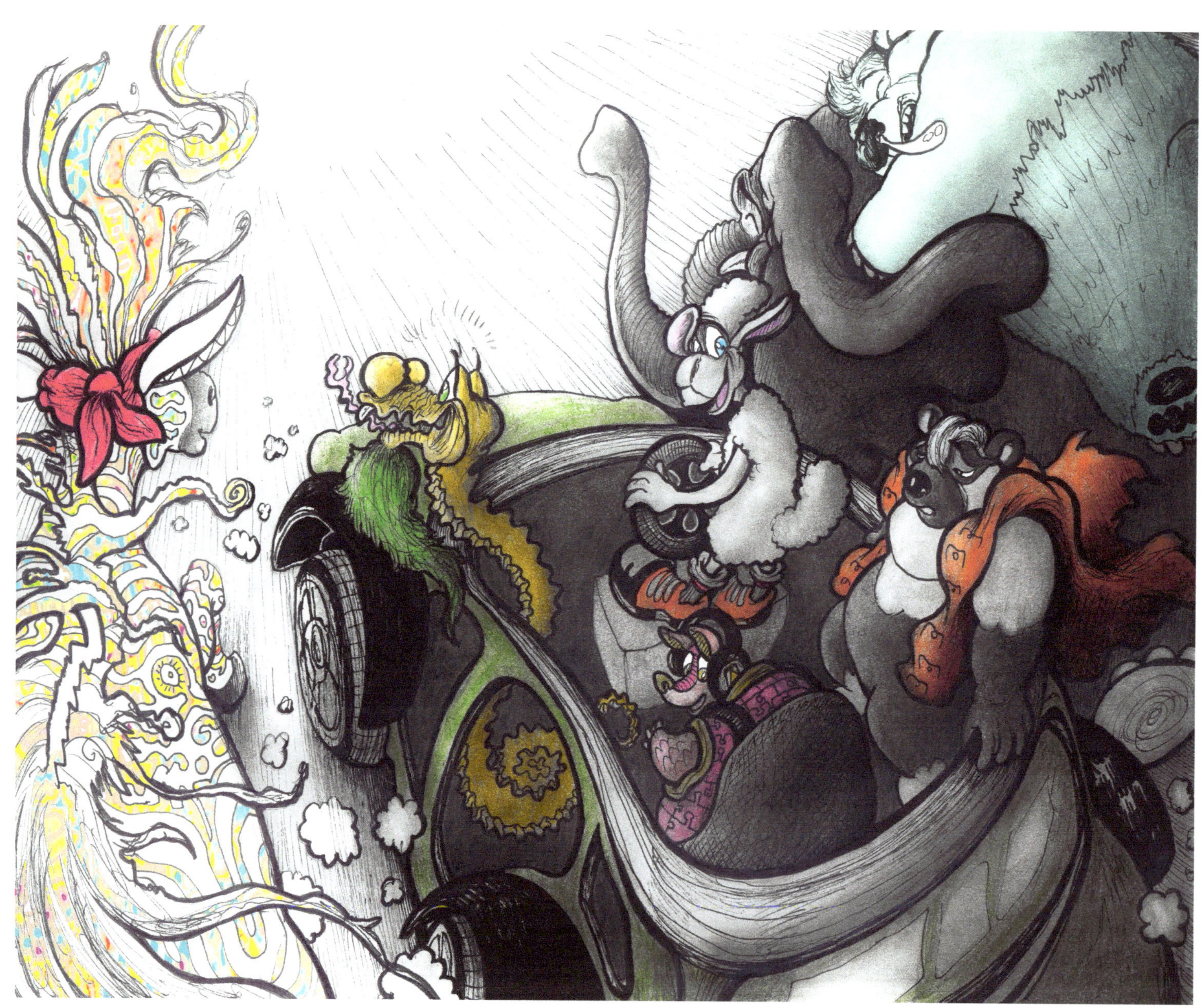

When they finally reached the hilltop they saw Eli's Elephant den a little
ways ahead,
However there was a raging river running through valley that they
feared they couldn't tread.
The jeep did not float, so they would have to swim across instead,
But the river looked scary, and the water was deeper than their head!

Just then a flash of feathers went sprinting by,
And, although it looked like a bird, this creature couldn't fly!
"Hey, wait for us," Yeshie yelled out to the speed-demon in reply,
But the long-legged bird just kept running—he refused to comply.

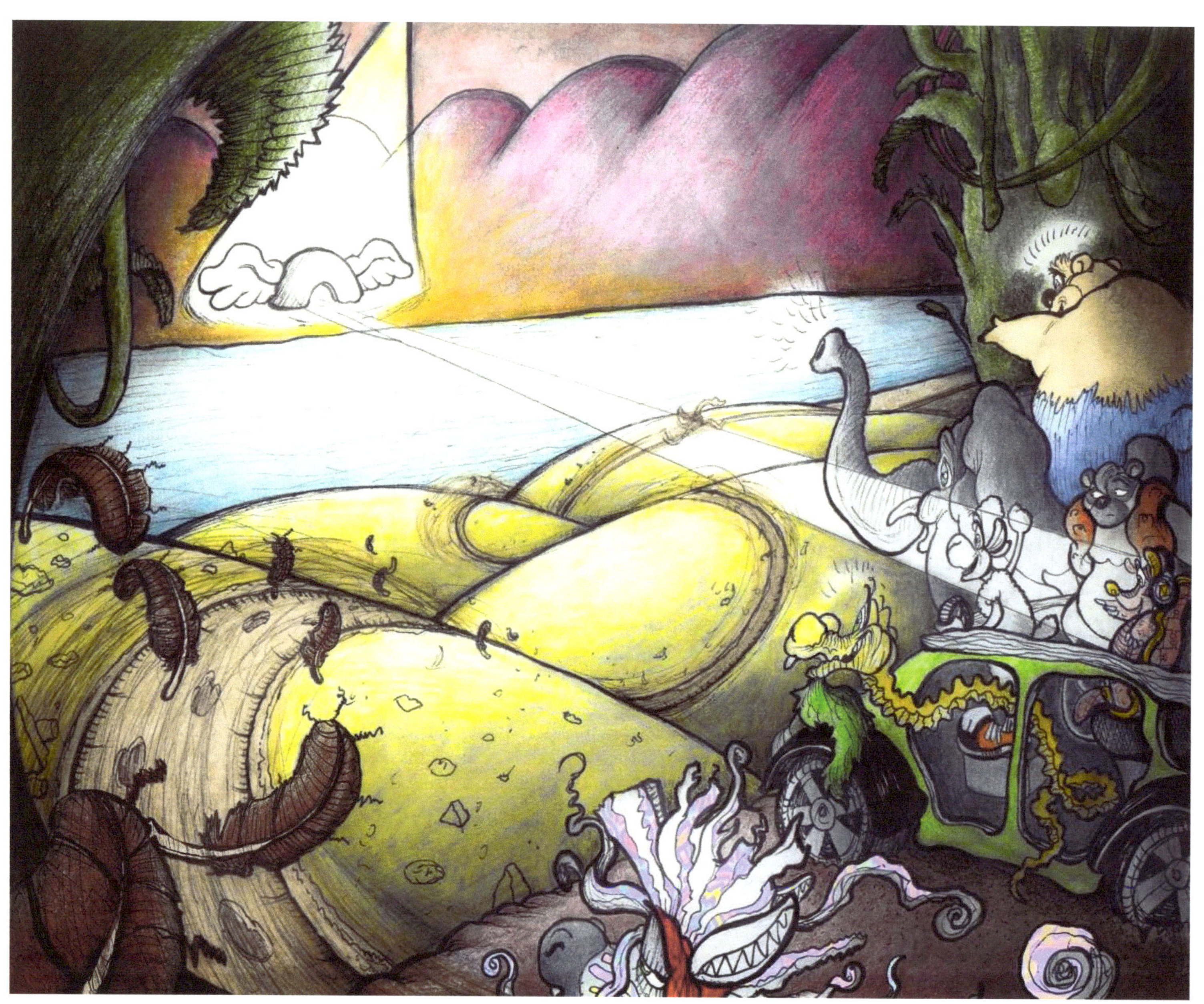

"Sorry but I cannot pause—I have to count my steps and wash my hands.
You see, their are germs in the jungle, all over the ground upon which you stand!"
"Germs?!" Eli the elephant said, as he looked downward at the sand."
"Yes. Germs!" the bobbing-headed bird shouted, before he turned away and ran.

They followed in his footsteps, hoping he might show them the way,
To get across the river, before they lost the light of day.
When the group finally caught the creature, it was as true as he did say,
He was washing his winged-hands with a bar of soap made out of clay.

"Excuse us Mr. Bird — we do not mean to seem rude,
But we need to find a way across the river, and you look like a pretty savvy dude!"
The tall and tidy feathered figure looked up and seemed amused,
"My name is Oscar—the Obsessive Compulsive Ostrich—and a solution I'll give you."

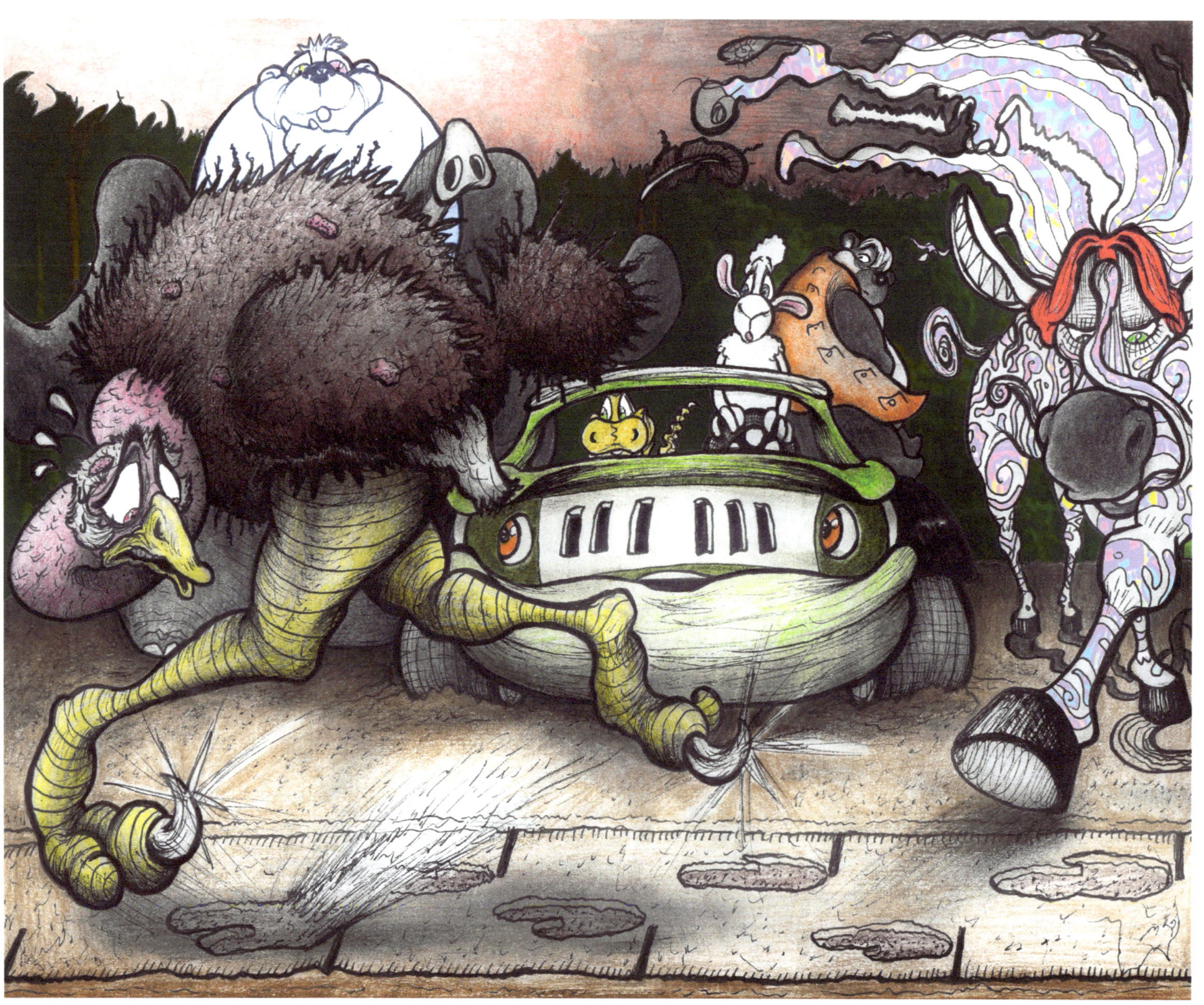

"Obsessive compulsive?" Eli repeated the strange words in the form of a question.
"Yes, it means that I fixate on certain routines, and, as for your query,
I have a suggestion!
Just watch my feet—toenails tidy and neat—and I will teach you an important lesson."
Then Oscar's legs started spinning, and with a flash the obsessive ostrich made quite the impression!

Although he could not fly, Oscar fast spinning legs skimmed across the water's surface,
Causing Eli and Anna to cheer; however, poor Yeshie got a little nervous.
Yeshie's short-sheep legs didn't move very fast and he feared sinking like a soggy clown in a circus.
The sheep had never learned to swim and, to that end, he spent his life away from the water on purpose.

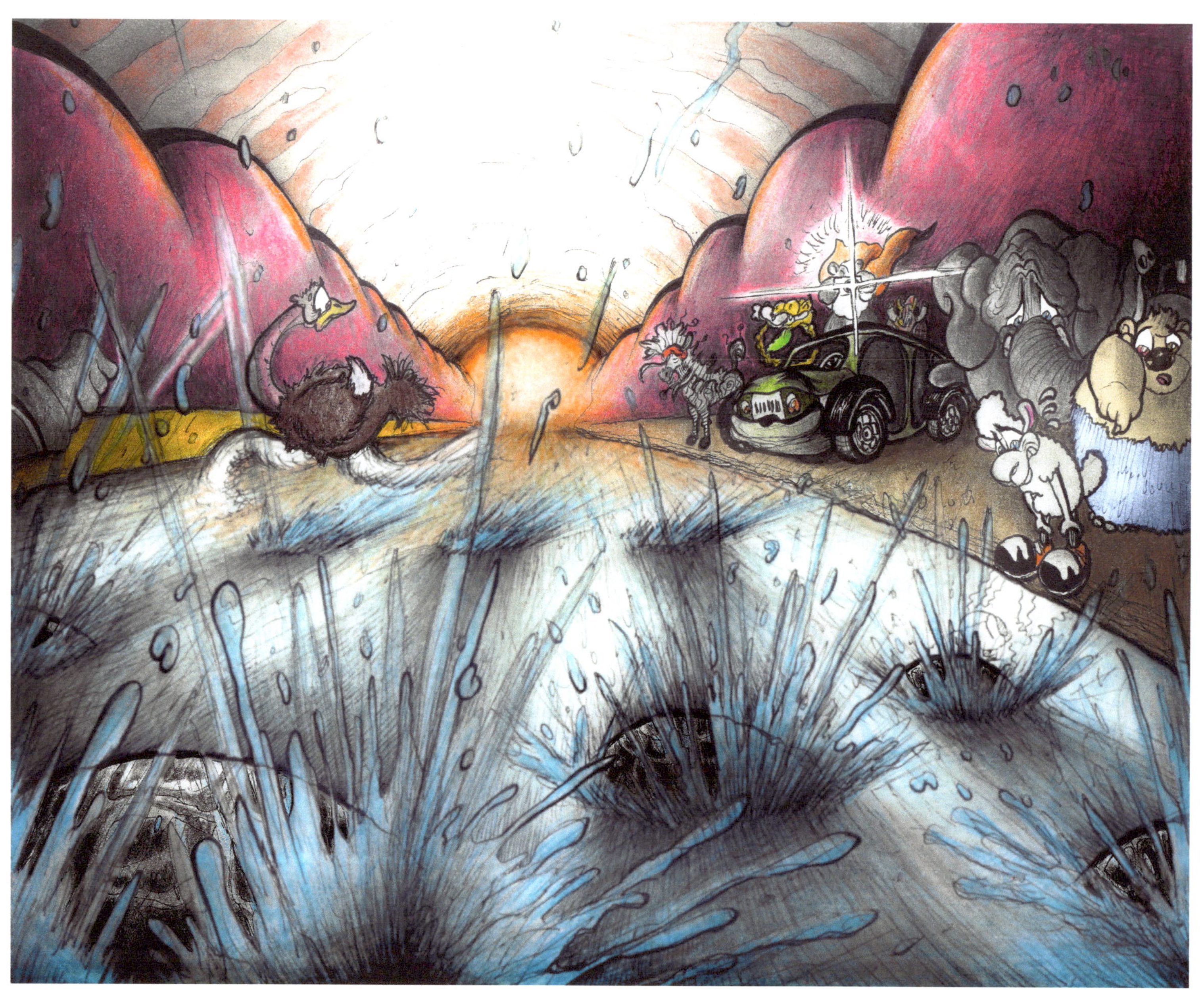

The sun had almost set and the friends were oh so close,
To Eli's den, but the rapids of the river were a bit too scary and
verbose.
But to the surprise of the armadillo, elephant, zebra, panda, bear and
Yeshie, their host,
A big round rock rose up from the rushing river, like a ghost!

At first there was just one, but one turned into five,
And the stones formed a path across the river on which the great
green jeep could drive!
The animals cheered as their journey had been revived,
But "Wait!" Eli exclaimed: "Those rocks look to be alive!"

As sure as the elephant spoke, one of the rocks grew a head and four feet,
And crawled out from the blue water that flowed so wide and deep.
The safariing squad stood in shock without a peep,
Until the rock yawned and said: "I'm Trevor, the traumatized tortoise,
and you awoke me from my sleep.

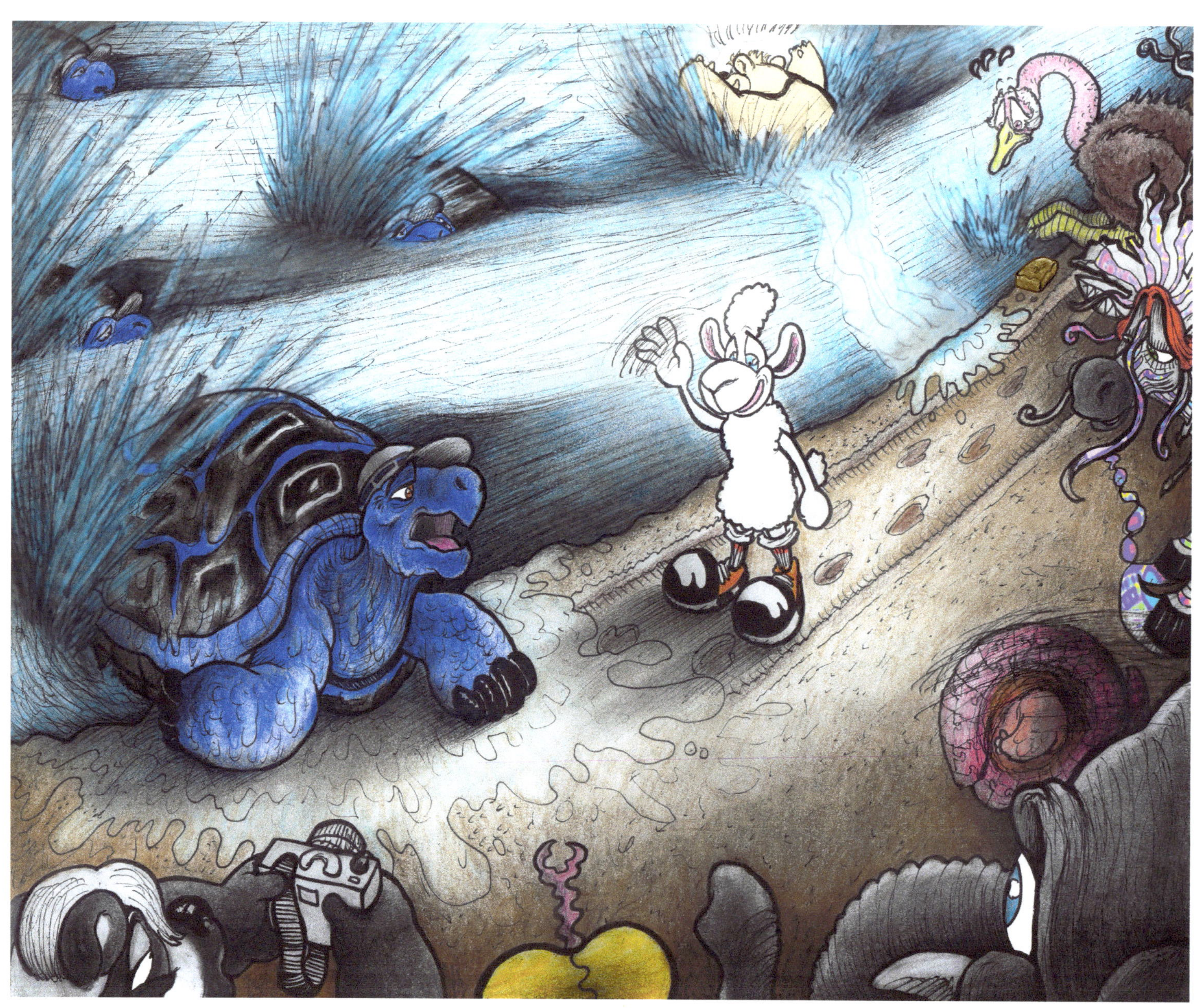

"Sorry Mr. Tortoise, we didn't mean to wake you from your dream,
But we need your help crossing the river," said the elephant as the
turtle studied the safariing team."
"Its okay," said the turtle, "these days I have more nightmares it'd seem,
So I am happy to be awake and glad to help you all cross the stream!"

"Nightmares?" Ana asked of the traumatized-tortoise,
"Unfortunately so, Mrs. Zebra—and they make me quite nervous.
You see, a long time ago my turtle friends and I served in the military
service,
And the violence we saw gave us Post-Traumatic Stress Disorders."

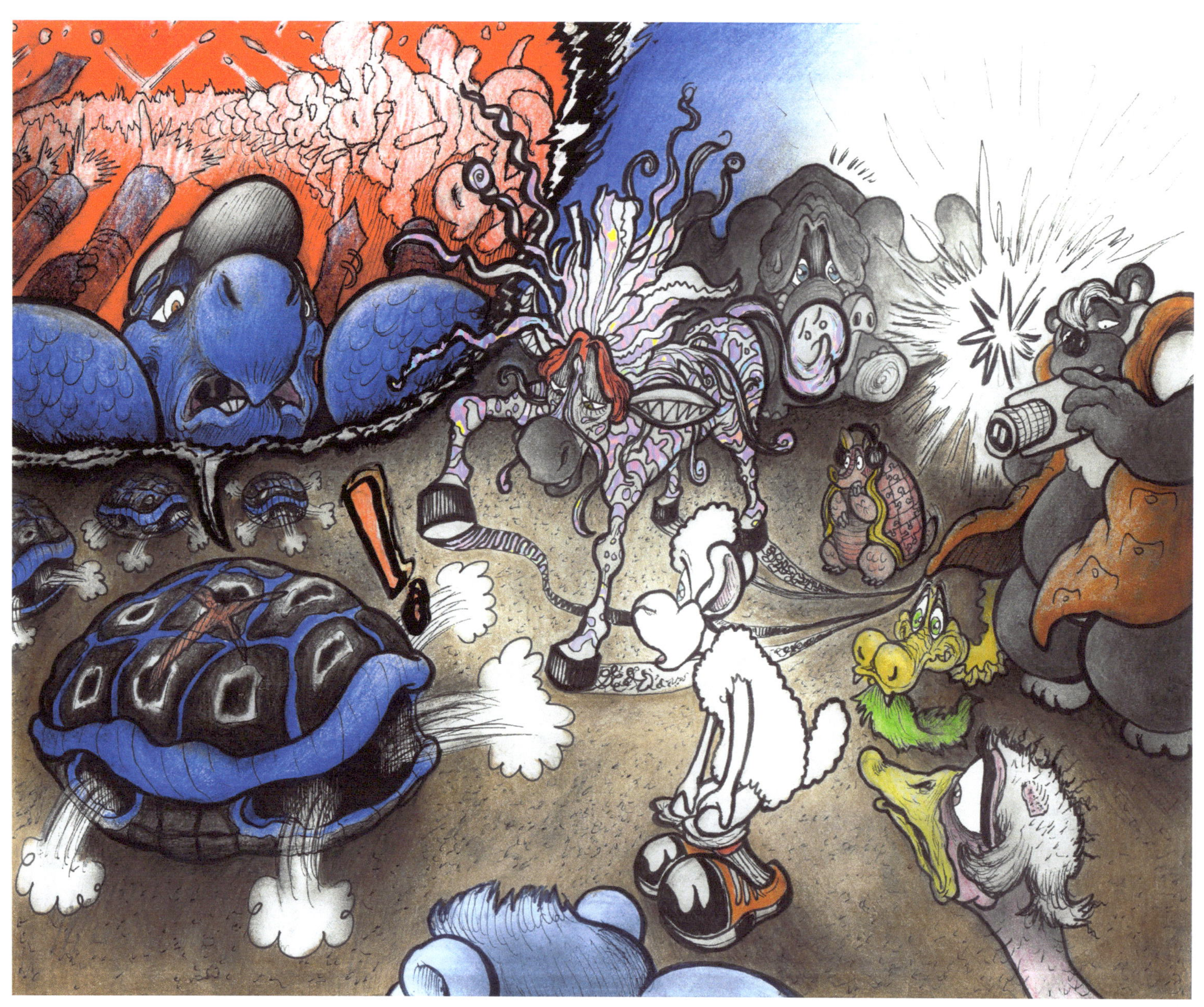

"We sure hate to hear that, no one likes to see fighting."
But Ana's words of support was interrupted by a flash of lightening.
Trevor's head disappeared into his shell at the sighting,
Loud sounds and bright lights were far too frightening.

"Its okay," said the zebra, "that was only the flash,
Of a camera that Patrick the Panda had stashed."
Since there was no lightening, there'd be no thunderous crash,
Just a portrait of the posse so the memory of the moment would last.

Trevor sure was relieved and willing to lend a shell,
The group of new friends who seemed super swell!
So he called together his Tortoise team with the sound of a bell,
And they formed a bridge to the den which Eli did dwell.

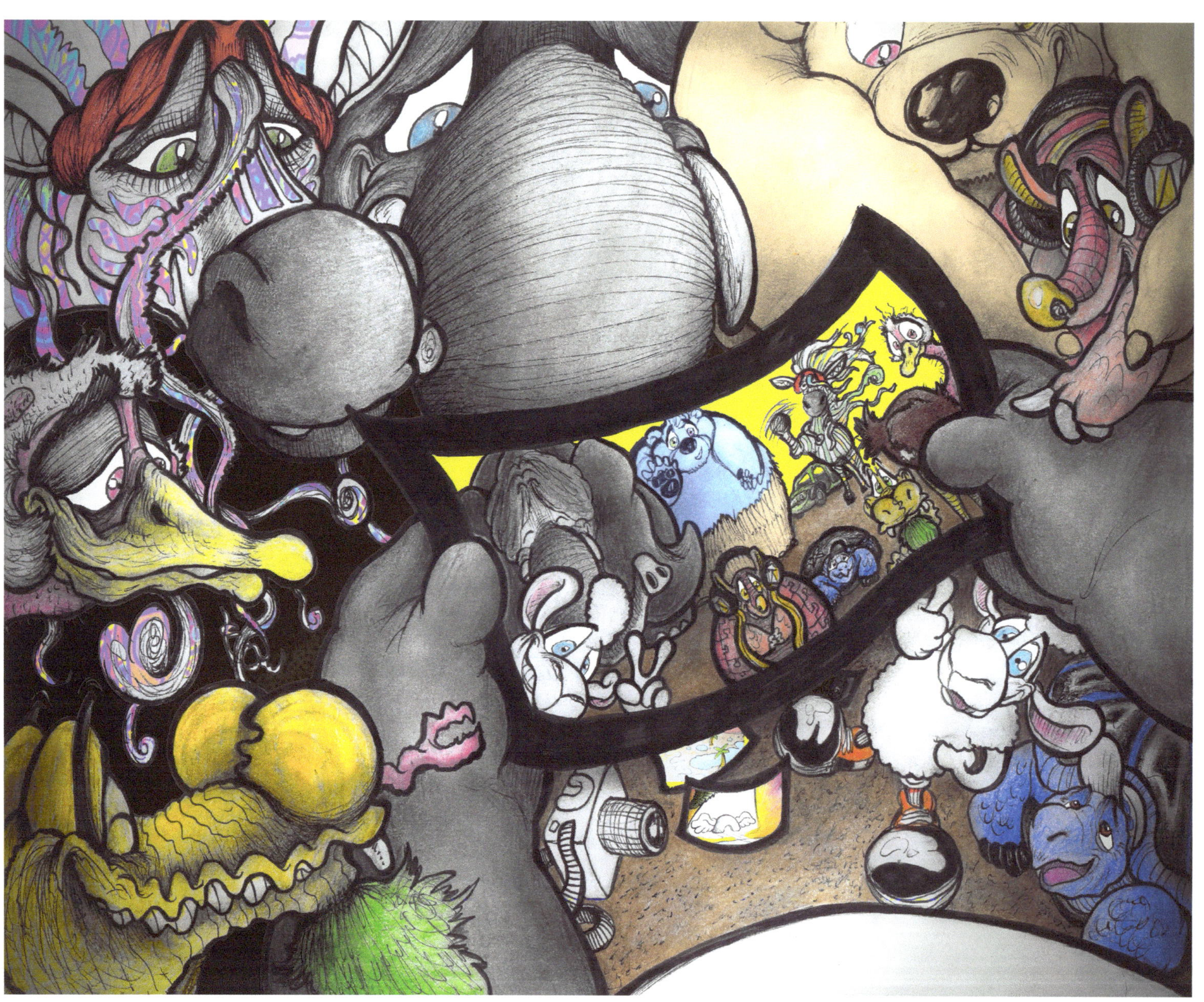

And with that the elephant, sheep, and bi-polar bear...
And Panda and zebra, with black and white hair,
All cheered and held hands as they skipped through the air,
Across tortoise shell-stepping stones, over the river in pairs.

They finally had made it to the elephant's enormous size home,
And Eli thanked them all with a mighty elephant-sized groan.
From savanna to jungle the diverse bunch had roamed,
Because together they could do what none of them could do alone!

The End.

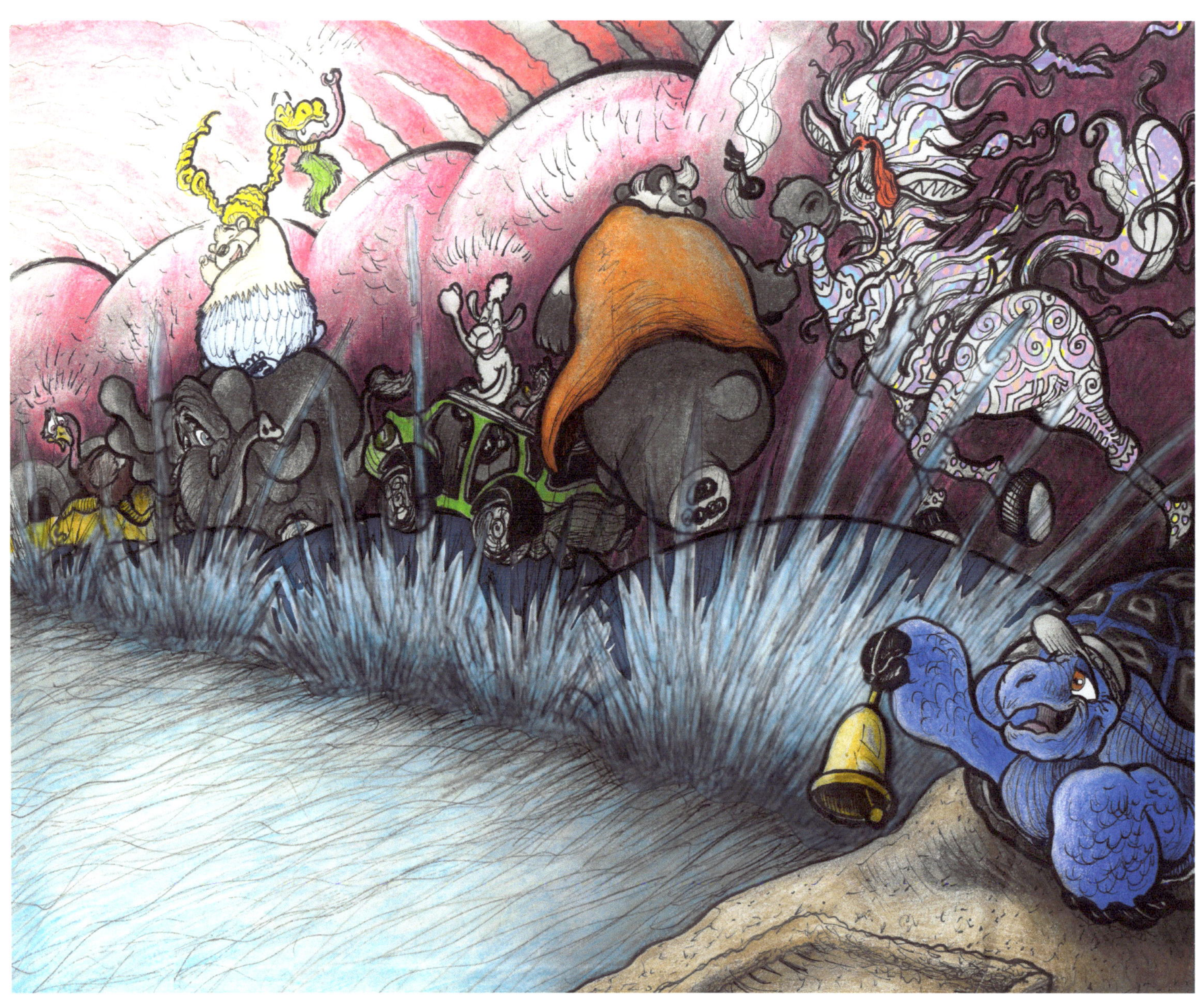

Salty Sheep is a movement calling us to engage in deliberative & interactive journeys, or 'wanderings' that utilize recreation as a means of breaking down sociological, economic, situational, cultural and faith divisions. In less words, we strive to promote the "POWER OF PLAY" in the cultivation of a more cohesive and fun community! Stay up to date with new books, fun ideas, events and all of our playful purity at www.saltysheep.org, and come surf, sail, garden, pray and play with us in Santa Cruz California anytime. Salty Sheep is a socially inclusive initiative that values the intrinsic potential, 'special gifts' and unique beauty of all faith, ethnic and social affiliations. In other words, we don't do black or white too well; thus have been deemed the Rainbow Sheep of the pasture—not afraid to question, doubt, explore, and wander this world with you at our side!

About the Author:

Rev. Ryan 'Mango' Althaus, known in Santa Cruz as the 'Pastor of Play," has spent the past several decades working intensively alongside various socially misperceived populations. His undergraduate work in English education and theology led to a master's degree in Divinity with a focus on world religious philosophy. You can find more of his writings and learn about his coaching practice by visiting, www.thesurfingMango.com. Ryan is also a licensed Captain who regularly hosts church on his sailing catamaran, the Minister of Interfaith Relations for the Santa Cruz Unitarian Universalist Fellowship, and the regional Hunger Inclusion affiliate for the National Presbyterian Church (USA).